T0171439

The Slim Book of Health Pearls

The Perfect Prescription

SHELDON COHEN M.D.FACP
MEGAN GODWIN HEALTH AND EXERCISE SCIENCE

iUniverse, Inc.
Bloomington

The Slim Book of Health Pearls
The Perfect Prescription

The information, ideas, and suggestions in this book are not intended as a substitute for professional medical advice. Before following any suggestions contained in this book, you should consult your personal physician. Neither the author nor the publisher shall be liable or responsible for any loss or damage allegedly arising as a consequence of your use or application of any information or suggestions in this book.

iUniverse books may be ordered through booksellers or by contacting:

iUniverse
1663 Liberty Drive
Bloomington, IN 47403
www.iuniverse.com
1-800-Authors (1-800-288-4677)

Because of the dynamic nature of the Internet, any Web addresses or links contained in this book may have changed since publication and may no longer be valid. The views expressed in this work are solely those of the author and do not necessarily reflect the views of the publisher, and the publisher hereby disclaims any responsibility for them.

Any people depicted in stock imagery provided by Thinkstock are models, and such images are being used for illustrative purposes only.

Certain stock imagery © Thinkstock.

ISBN: 978-1-4502-9616-8 (pbk)
ISBN: 978-1-4502-9617-5 (ebk)

Printed in the United States of America

iUniverse rev. date: 2/4/2011

THIS BOOK IS DEDICATED TO

GAIL COHEN
A DEVOTED EXERCISER, GRANDMOTHER,
MOTHER AND DAUGHTER

AND

CARLY GODWIN
WHO PREPARED A BEAUTIFUL POWER POINT
PRESENTATION BASED ON THIS BOOK

WE LOVE YOU BOTH INFINITY

This book offers advice on how to promote long-term health. The perfect prescription in the subtitle is EXERCISE and the authors will discuss the many different ailments that benefit from this simple act. As always, consult a physician before starting any exercise program. Exercise may often equal or surpass the benefits of medication. Each person may have a different set of unique needs. How to start and evolve any exercise program is best accomplished with physician guidance. The book is thin—a quick read. The authors hope that the benefit accrued will be well worth the short amount of time spent with this book.

First, the authors will discuss the benefits and the risks of prescription drugs. The idea is to get a better understanding of how prescription drugs affect patients, and, most importantly, the patient's role in preventing the many medical errors that can result from the simple act of writing, dispensing and taking a prescription. With the coming healthcare changes to be, it becomes more important than ever that each patient take an active and leading role in their medical care.

A prescription drug is a medicine used to treat a symptom or an illness or prevent an illness from occurring. The government regulates all prescription drugs and only medical professionals including physicians, dentists, nurse practitioners, psychologists, optometrists and veterinarians can prescribe them. This is nothing new.

A medical professor at the University Of Illinois College Of Medicine once said to his class of students, "Just remember, medicines are simply controlled poisons. If taken in excess, they can kill. Even if taken as directed they can cause harm, but more often than not, they are little miracles, providing relief and controlling or curing disease. Treat them with great respect and use them only when necessary, because they all have the potential for side-effects and, at times, those side-effects can be serious."

As the population increases, there is a greater demand for prescription drugs of all categories. Pain medications have the potential to cause addiction and abuse. These deleterious effects result in reluctance to prescribe pain medication because of the possibility of serious or fatal consequences—as well as the specter of malpractice which looms like a cloud over the medical community.

When healthcare professionals give patients a prescription for the first time, they can never know what the reaction will be. Side effects can occur, even with a single pill—and sometimes the side effects can have severe consequences. Here following are two real-life examples that reflect rare but serious side effects:

1) A middle-aged healthy man, Mr. L., injured his shoulder. He took an unprescribed medication for the pain he was experiencing. One day after taking the medicine, he went to the hospital emergency room complaining of weakness, loss of appetite, nausea and vomiting. He felt he was "dehydrated" and it dawned upon him that he had not passed any urine for "a long time." When asked if he was on any medicines he said no, but his wife pointed out that he had taken one of her rheumatoid arthritis pills for his shoulder. His wife—who had severe rheumatoid arthritis—was on a non-steroidal anti-inflammatory medicine. Blood studies on Mr. L. revealed evidence of uremia (kidney failure). Prior to this incident, he was perfectly healthy describing himself as "Never sick a day in my life." The significance of his uremia became evident. He developed acute kidney failure from taking merely *one* of his wife's pills. What happened was a very rare complication of the non-steroidal anti-inflammatory class of drugs—kidney shutdown. He underwent acute renal dialysis treatments and made a full recovery.

2) A patient received numerous medications after undergoing heart surgery. Prior to the surgery, his blood count was normal. As expected, the surgery lowered his blood count. The blood loss during surgery should have resolved and gone back to normal within weeks of the operation, but it did not; it continued downward. His physician sent the patient to a

hematologist who recommended that he have a bone marrow biopsy. The patient decided to hold off on this procedure while he did his own personal research. He went on the internet and studied his medications, all of whom had the rare potential to cause anemia. He thought, could this be it? Is one of the medications causing this? After getting approval from his personal doctor, he discontinued the last medication prescribed for his prostate symptoms. He repeated the blood count after a month. Much to his relief the count was back to normal. He had a very rare side effect of a medication prescribed for his enlarged prostate. He saved himself a bone marrow biopsy, and his hematologist learned something too. This case is an excellent example of a patient who took responsibility for his health.

Remember that the billions of prescriptions carry with them the small potential for error that could be serious or fatal. Here are some measures patients can take to safeguard their health by preventing medication errors:

1) When a physician or other healthcare provider writes a prescription, be certain that it is easy to read. If not, a pharmacist may have the same trouble reading the prescription. Ask that the prescription is rewritten, or at the very least, that it be spelled out in writing.

Sound-alike medications with similar spelling can be confused. The busy pharmacist could misread the medication or confuse it with a medicine that has a similar sounding name resulting in dispensing the wrong medication.

Different manufacturers make generic medications with a dissimilar appearance and this could cause the patient to become confused. The patient needs to clarify the issue before taking the unfamiliar medication.

Pharmacists fill many prescriptions and pharmacy

technicians often have an excessive workload. Failure of the pharmacist to check everything the technician does can also cause prescription errors. Patients must double-check this complicated process.

2) Patient should bring a written list of all medications prescribed by every physician they may have seen to every doctor visit. Some larger clinics and University Medical Centers will have the full medication list printed out for evaluation at each visit. If the physician is not doing this, then patients can help themselves and the physician by coming to the office visit prepared with a full medication list including vitamins, herbs and dietary supplements. Patients can even brown-bag the medicines and bring them along.

Patients allergic to any medication should wear a wristband, which identifies the offending agent or agents. Patients must make physicians aware of any medication allergies, so the information can occupy a prominent part of the patient record.

Patients given a prescription must know the following:
- What is the medicine and what does it do?
- How long should it be taken and at what intervals?
- What are some side effects to watch for?
- Are there any potential drug-food or medication-medication interactions that may cause a problem by enhancing or hindering the action of the prescription?
- What are some activities that the patient should avoid?

Patients should not ignore the written information dispensed with each medication. Read it with care. If there are any questions, it is much better to ask than to take a risk.

3) A hospitalized patient who receives an unfamiliar appearing medication must not take it until the patient has clarified the issue. This is critical in the era of generics drugs when the same generic made by different pharmaceutical companies have a dissimilar appearance.

Once checked into a hospital, an alert patient must continue to be aware of their medication as well as their general health status. When transferring a patient from one unit to another while in the hospital medical errors are prone to occur. Case in point:

A woman was walking her dog on a residential side street and noticed a neighbor lying unconscious on her garage floor. She rushed in, was unable to revive her, and called the paramedics who transported the unconscious woman to the closest hospital emergency department. Examination revealed a seventy-five-year-old with a bruised head. An emergency CT scan of the head revealed a subdural hematoma (collection of blood under the brain covering). This hematoma was very small, so her physicians elected watchful waiting rather than surgery. The patient regained consciousness, but was very restless and agitated, a state that persisted over the next few days. She also had some difficulty in walking, lost strength in one of her extremities and required the use of a walker. The patient was rational, but stated that she was jumping out of her skin. This persisted until the physician prescribed a tranquilizer. The anxiety resolved, but the patient then became confused and disoriented. This worried her physician who ordered further tests thinking that perhaps the hematoma had enlarged, or other cerebral pathology had developed, or there were yet undiagnosed medical problems; there were no new findings.

Now turning his attention to the tranquilizer, the physician stopped it on the chance that it was the cause of the sudden confusion and disorientation. Within two days, the patient's confusion and disorientation was resolved.

All this time there was a delay in transferring the patient to the rehabilitation unit, because to do so requires a clear mind and a cooperative patient, neither of which was possible while symptoms were present. She improved, was transferred and her care was taken over by a different physician. She started rehabilitation, but progress became impossible because confusion and disorientation returned. They called the patient's hospital physician to tell him what happened. In the meantime, progress was not possible for a full week due to an altered mental state. When the hospital physician arrived, he discovered why the patient had relapsed. Somehow—and no one could tell him how—the medication that he had discontinued and that had caused her confusion and disorientation had been restarted. Someone must have ignored or missed the transfer instructions. This medical error caused considerable delay, added to the cost, set back the patient's progress and could have resulted in serious consequences. This situation is a good example of how imperative it is that there are no mistakes made, and that the patient should take charge of their health if they are mentally capable.

There are some things a patient cannot have total control over, but should verify that the nurse in charge knows. For example: If a hospitalized patient receives intravenous medication, the nurse in charge should know how long the intravenous is supposed to drip before it runs out and should tell the patient. If not informed, the patient should ask.

Before dispensing medication of any kind, the nurse must identify every patient. Failure to do this will not only lead to medication errors, but also testing errors, transfusion errors, and possibly the discharge of infants to the wrong family.

As can be seen from the aforementioned examples, the simple act of receiving a prescription is fraught with the possibility of unwanted and untoward events. Again, recall what a professor of medicine said, "Just remember, medicines are controlled poisons; if taken in excess, they can kill. Even if taken as directed they can cause harm, but more often than not, they are little miracles, providing relief and controlling or curing disease. Treat them with great respect and use them only when necessary, because they all have the potential for side-effects and, at time, those side-effects can be serious."

This may soon change as we enter the exciting era of **personalized medicine:** tailoring treatment to a patient's genetic profile. Personalized medicine, known as pharmacogenomics or pharmacogenetics, is the study of how the inherited variations in individual genes affect how the body processes and responds to medicines. The idea behind it is that once genetic variations are identified, patients will be matched to a particular medication and then as the name implies develop a personalized approach to medicine. The day may come when gene variations will be determined enabling personalization of therapy. Will this eliminate the gamble inherent in writing prescriptions? That is the hope. The result will be superior medication choices with safer dosing options. Through clinical trials, drug companies will be able to develop safer drugs by excluding those who have the genetic variation, which will cause an adverse interaction with the drug. Reduced healthcare costs could result by reducing the number of deaths and hospitalizations from adverse drug reactions. We are in the early stages. The future holds great promise.

Here is another principle to ponder.

Before release of a medication, it must undergo a rigid period of testing for proof of effectiveness. This is a lengthy process estimated to take eight years through three phases.

Phase 1 studies involve twenty to eighty either healthy volunteers or patients. Researchers study mechanisms of action and side effects of the drug in humans.

Phase 2 involves clinical trials on several hundred patients with a specific medical condition. Its purpose is to determine the drug's efficacy and side effects.

Phase 3 studies provide additional information on the drug's efficacy, involves thousands of patients, more information about side effects and allows scientists to extrapolate the results to the general population.

Once these three phases are completed, the drug sponsor will make a formal application to the Food and Drug Administration (FDA) who determines if the drug is safe and effective and the benefits outweigh the risk.

If agreed by all experts concerned, the FDA will release the drug to the general population.

Now the true test starts. Many thousands, perhaps millions will benefit from the drug. However, there will be those who may suffer serious consequences. One needs only to watch television to understand. Hardly a day goes by that there is not a class action lawsuit advertised by one law firm or another inviting all those harmed to join the suit. Some of these drugs have been available to the public for twenty or thirty years. This exemplifies that the true test of a drug's efficacy is when the FDA releases the drug to the vast general population. This problem will continue to persist until and if personalized medicine ever comes to pass. There are three medications currently available to genetic determination (personalized medicine) as to whether or not a patient will react unfavorably. This knowledge will be available to prescribing physicians allowing them to determine in advance whether to prescribe the drug. Let us hope there will be many more drugs available in the future.

To establish an important general principle that applies to all prescription medication, and before discussion of The Perfect Prescription, it will be helpful to learn about a common and important medicine—the STATIN group of drugs. Their purpose is to lower cholesterol and they have revolutionized the treatment of coronary artery and other vascular disease and have other important indications.

THE STATINS:

Cholesterol is a fatty substance used to form cell membranes and some hormones. Fatty substances like cholesterol cannot dissolve in the blood stream. When combined with a protein they become soluble. There are three types of lipoproteins: low-density lipoproteins (LDL), high-density lipoproteins (HDL), and very low-density lipoproteins (VLDL). Each type contains a mixture of cholesterol, protein and triglyceride (fatty substance). LDL contains the highest amount of cholesterol, HDL contains the highest amount of protein and VLDL contains the highest amount of triglyceride. The total cholesterol is a combination of the three forms LDL plus HDL plus VLDL. There is no easy way to measure the VLDL, and that is why laboratories do not report it. It is a percentage of the triglyceride. Laboratories calculate total cholesterol by formula: total cholesterol = LDL + HDL + $1/5^{th}$ of the triglyceride (if the triglyceride is less than 400).

Normal total cholesterol is under 150 mg/dl (milligrams per deciliter).

LDL Cholesterol is the principle carrier of cholesterol in the blood. If the concentration of LDL is too high, it deposits in arteries as plaques, causing the arteries to block up and result in a heart attack or stroke. "Bad cholesterol" is the perfect name for LDL. The body acquires cholesterol in two ways: ingestion and liver production. The liver produces all the cholesterol one requires meaning that it is not essential to ingest cholesterol. Cholesterol is present in meat and is absent in fruits and vegetables. Total cholesterol intake should be limited. Besides cholesterol, saturated fats and Trans fats also cause plaque.

Normal LDL cholesterol is less than100 mg/dl. In a higher risk cardiac patient with other important risk factors, the goal is as low as 70 mg/dl.

HOW TO LOWER AN ELEVATED LDL CHOLSTEROL
1. Eat a Low-saturated fat, low cholesterol diet plan that avoids weight gain. The plan should not have more than seven percent of calories from saturated fat and should have less than 200 milligrams of cholesterol per day.
2. Weight management: lose weight if overweight.
3. Exercise at least thirty minutes every day. This is important for those with an elevated triglyceride and a large waist measurement (more than 40 inches in men and 35 inches in women).
4. Eat at least two servings of soluble fiber per day (oats, fruits, vegetables, legumes).
5. Medication, principally the statin family of drugs, may be necessary.

HDL Cholesterol constitutes about thirty percent of the blood cholesterol. HDL cholesterol removes excess cholesterol from artery blockages and thus slows down the growth. It is for this reason that HDL is "good cholesterol," so the higher the better. Exercise raises HDL cholesterol. Smoking and excess weight are detrimental to healthy HDL levels.
Normal is greater than 40mg/dl.

HOW TO INCREASE A LOW HDL CHOLESTEROL

1. Exercise at least four days per week and increase to safe prescribed levels for twenty to thirty minutes at a time under physician supervision.
2. Lose weight.
3. Stop smoking.
4. Stop consuming Trans fats as much as possible
5. Discontinue drinking more than one or two drinks of alcohol per day
6. Eat at least two servings per day of soluble fiber.
7. Eat monounsaturated fats (peanut butter, avocado oil, canola oil)
8. Consume Omega 3 fatty acids (present in fish and flax)
9. Consume Niacin, which is found in liver, poultry, fish, whole grains, nuts
10. Medication, as prescribed by a physician

Triglyceride

The largest percentage of fat in the diet and in fatty tissues is in the form of triglyceride. Triglycerides in the blood plasma are derived from fats eaten in foods and are made in the body from other energy sources like carbohydrates. The carbohydrates convert to triglycerides and are stored in fat cells if not used by tissues. Hormones regulate triglyceride's release from the fat cells for use in energy generation. Elevation of triglycerides correlates with a higher risk for heart attack and stroke. This is truer if other risk factors are present such as obesity or diabetes.

Normal is less than 150 mg/dl.

HOW TO DECREASE AN ELEVATED TRIGLYCERIDE

Lose weight
Discontinue the consumption of alcohol
Reduce Trans fats, saturated fat and cholesterol in the diet
Exercise

Reduce carbohydrates in the diet
Consume Omega 3 fatty acids found in fish or commercially in capsules
Limit sugar intake to aid in the prevention of type II diabetes

To reduce cholesterol that will not come down with the above life style changes, the statin drugs are "little miracles." They are very effective. Many millions are reaping their benefits. As already discussed, they have changed the therapy of coronary artery disease. However, as with all medications they are not risk free. Drug companies that manufacture statin drugs have added a warning: "Unexplained muscle pain and weakness could be a symptom of a rare but serious side effect and should be reported to your doctor right away."

The muscle pain and weakness is a result of muscle breakdown in the body (rhabdomyolysis) caused by the statin drug. The kidneys must eliminate the muscle breakdown products and they may overload the kidneys resulting in kidney failure that could result in death. The other major symptom of rhabdomyolysis is red, dark or cola colored urine. There have been thirty-three hundred cases of rhabdomyolysis reported between 1990 and 2002. This figure, as bad as it is for those afflicted, represents a very tiny percentage of the millions who take the drug, so the benefit-risk ratio is acceptable.
One to five percent of those who take the statin drugs will experience some muscle pain.

Statins may also cause a peripheral neuropathy—damage to the nerves that may result in muscle weakness, numbness, tingling, or burning sensations. These symptoms may be rapid or slow in onset and escape recognition. In extreme cases, neuropathy can lead to death.

Some patients that are prescribed statins experience memory loss and an inability to concentrate and worry that they are developing Alzheimer's disease. The memory loss is more than patient perception; family members confirm this to the patient's physician. (However, a new study suggests that one of the statin drugs lowers the risk of Alzheimer's disease and Parkinson's disease).

On the other hand, the statin drugs have anti-inflammatory and anti-angiogenesis (anti blood vessel growth) affects. This opens up new areas of potential therapeutic benefit that are under study at this time.

Therefore, it is clear that with all prescribed medications—and over-the-counter medications—there are benefits and there are risks. The benefit to risk evaluation is a joint responsibility of the physician and the patient. The final decision to take or not to take the medication, as always, rests in the patient's hands.

Now we will discuss *The Perfect Prescription*

"Better to hunt in fields for health unbought,
Than fee the doctor for a nauseous draught.
The wise, for cure, on exercise depend;
God never made his work for man to mend."

John Dryden
1628-1687

Yes, that is right—The Perfect Prescription is exercise. First, let us see what a biblical scholar advised:

Maimonides (Rambam), the great Torah scholar, philosopher and physician of the 12th century, said,

"As long as a person exercises and exerts himself...sickness does not befall him and his strength increases... But one who is idle and does not exercise...even if he eats healthy foods and maintains healthy habits, all his days will be of ailment and his strength will diminish."

The Rambam defined exercise as "vigorous or gentle movement, or a combination of the two, which increases one's breathing rate." Doesn't this sound like brisk walking, jogging, swimming, or biking?

With regular exercise, one will feel better, have more energy, strengthen the immune system, avoid illness, maintain ideal weight, sleep better and live longer. These benefits are open to all regardless of age. There has never been a therapeutic agent that could equal it, and there never will be. It affects multiple organ systems. It is a miracle—and it is free!

We will now discuss the "abc's" of the benefits of exercise.

ALZHEIMER'S DISEASE

Dementia: a partial or complete loss of mind. Dementia is a symptom that has many causes. A physician who sees a patient with dementia must first consider reversible causes, because the problem is amenable to correction.

Reversible or partially reversible causes include:
Head trauma
Infections of the brain (encephalitis) or brain covering (meningitis) secondary to many viruses including HIV, and bacteria and fungi
Benign or malignant brain tumors
Toxins including heavy metals (lead) and solvents
Diseases of the liver, pancreas or kidneys can disrupt the balance of body chemicals and electrolytes (salts)
Drugs, both legal (sleeping pills and tranquilizers) and illegal (cocaine and heroin)
Poor oxygenation caused by heart failure and/or lung failure
An increase of cerebrospinal fluid (hydrocephalus) either within or around the brain;
Hormone imbalances
Nutritional deficiencies especially B vitamins
Alcoholism

Irreversible causes:
Vascular dementia caused by many small strokes due to hardening of the arteries
Dementia may be part of late-stage Parkinson's disease
Huntington's disease, an inherited brain disorder, may lead to dementia

Lewy body dementia caused by abnormal deposits of protein in the brain
Creuzfeld-Jacob disease caused by infectious agents called prions that infect and kill brain cells
Picks disease, a rarer type of dementia involving only the frontal and temporal part of the brain (frontotemporal dementia)
In addition, the final cause of irreversible dementia:

Alzheimer's disease.

Alois Alzheimer M.D. (1864-1915) was a German neuropsychiatrist who described a very unusual patient he first saw in 1901. He published his findings in 1906 from a postmortem examination of her brain *"eine eigenartige Erkrankung der Hirnrinde"* (a peculiar disease of the cerebral cortex). The patient was a woman in her fifties.

In those days, people did not live as long as they do today. There was the common senility of old age, and there was the rare younger case similar to Alzheimer's patient who became more and more disoriented, suffered increasing memory impairment and lost the ability to read and to write.

We now live much longer. Alzheimer's disease can strike victims as young as fifty. The incidence increases with time so that fifty percent of us by age eighty-five have developed the disease. There are more than 4.5 million Americans afflicted. Can we do anything to prevent it? By 2050, this figure will grow to 13.2 million. Current medications are not curative, but can slow the progression of the memory deterioration and cognitive impairment.

Studies have demonstrated a decreased risk of Alzheimer's disease through physical exercise done on a regular basis, at least three times per week and one half hour per day.

Current research demonstrates that exercise might shift the brain's metabolic pathways that break down the amyloid precursor protein and prevent the buildup of amyloid deposits that cause Alzheimer's disease.

Exercise is but one-way to forestall Alzheimer's disease. There are others:

Proper nutrition will reduce the risk of Alzheimer's disease:
1. Eat food low in cholesterol and saturated fats (heart healthy)
2. Eat food with a high level of omega-3 fatty acids that are beneficial to cell membranes
These foods include:
Coldwater fish such as trout, tuna, salmon, herring, and sardines
Canola oil, olive oil, peanut oil, flaxseed oil, green leafy vegetables
Brazil nuts, cashews, walnuts, pistachios, avocados
3. Eat foods that are high in antioxidants that protect the brain from free radical formation to reduce the risk of Alzheimer's disease. A free radical is an atom or group of atoms that has at least one unpaired electron and is therefore unstable and very reactive. Free radicals can damage cells and accelerate the progression of Alzheimer's disease as well as other age-related diseases.

Foods high in antioxidants include:
All types of berries
Dark-skinned fruits and vegetables such as beets, spinach, broccoli, brussel sprouts,
Eggplant, red bell peppers, beets, red grapes, oranges, cherries
4. Supplements such as a multivitamin including folic acid may help in Alzheimer's disease prevention. Research shows that those deficient in folic acid were three times more likely to develop Alzheimer's disease. Experts agree, however, that it is better to obtain supplements from food rather than from vitamin tablets.

Mental activity will reduce the risk of Alzheimer's disease

Remaining alert strengthens the connection between brain cells and can add more brain cells, contrary to the myth that new brain cells do not form in adults. To benefit from this finding one must commit to a lifetime of learning: the internet, educational TV, games, crossword puzzles, reading and writing. Recent research suggests that this will delay Alzheimer's, but once it breaks through, the disease will have a faster downhill course.

Social activity will reduce the risk of Alzheimer's disease

An active social life is good for the brain because it stimulates connections between brain cells. Social activity promotes use of parts of the brain that would otherwise remain idle. Good ways to remain socially active include working, volunteering, membership in book clubs or other clubs and traveling in groups. Always try learning new things; it becomes contagious and results in increasing alertness. Life will become more interesting and more brain cells will develop.

AEROBIC CAPACITY

Human beings are aerobic because we live and grow in an environment rich in oxygen. The aerobic capacity is the amount of work done in this environment and is built up by exercise when we use the muscles of our arms and legs over an extended period. The energy for this activity comes from oxygen in our atmosphere.

Aerobic capacity increases with exercises such as walking, jogging, any active sports, cycling and swimming. Other terms for aerobic capacity include aerobic power, maximal functional capacity, cardiorespiratory fitness, cardiovascular fitness and maximal oxygen uptake.

Aerobic capacity declines with age and this has substantial implications for quality of life in those who enjoy good health, but is of greater significance to those with chronic disease.

Some people's genes predispose them to Alzheimer's disease, but researchers have found that exercise has the power to change the structure of their brain and reduce their risk to a level similar to one with no genetic predisposition.

By increasing the body's ability to utilize oxygen, exercise promotes better health. Every organ system in the body benefits by the improved oxygen delivery.

BACK HEALTH AND FUNCTIONALITY

Low back pain, caused by muscle strain or injury, is very common in adults. As long as a physician confirms the diagnosis, a patient can embark upon self-treatment if there are no serious causes identified.

Fifty years ago, the recommendation for low back strain was bed rest. As it turned out this did nothing but delay recovery. Simple measures such as staying active, the use of ice and possibly nonprescription pain relievers pus avoiding those positions or movements that bring on greater pain is often all that is necessary.

As soon as the pain gets to a point that one is able, exercise will put the icing on the cake. Special equipment is not necessary. Exercises for the back, abdomen and legs are best. Your physician may want you to consult with a personal trainer or a physical therapist to find exercises that best suit your needs. They will ease pain, accelerate recovery, minimize the risk of future disability and prevent recurrences.

Case in point: physician A was the victim of repeated back sprains. He spoke to a fellow physician, B, who happened to be a black belt in one of the martial arts and suffered from repetitive back pain. The black belt's "Dogo Master" taught B six exercises that eliminated the problem. After B taught A, A has never had a recurrence of the severe back strains that had been so prevalent in the past.

BALANCE & COORDINATION

Falls are a significant problem for the elderly. By the time one reaches the age of forty, balance and coordination have begun to decline. The rate of decline is about one percent per year. However, even at that rate, the decline could be about thirty percent by the time one reaches age 70. In one who leads a sedentary existence this rate of decline is inevitable. The greater the loss of balance and coordination one experiences, the greater the risk of falls. Falls can have very deleterious effects—fractures and head injuries, both of which can cause death.

Much of this is preventable and all that is necessary is to exercise; and the time to start is at the age of forty.

First test balance and assess ability. Have an observer close by.

Stand in front of an open door. If necessary, use the doorframes for support. Once in position, lift one foot off the floor and place it behind you. Now see if it is possible to stand on one foot for one minute without the need of hand support. Do this also with the other foot. Once able to do stand for one minute it is time for the next exercise.

Do the same thing, but this time pick one foot up behind you and high enough so that your lower leg is parallel to the floor. Bend the knee of the other leg. This is more difficult than the first balance test. Keep practicing until standing this way for one minute on each leg. Then try the next tests with a helper:

This test has three parts:
1. Walk forward on the toes.
2. Walk forward on the heels.

3. Do a cross over walk. Walk sidewise, crossing the right foot over the left. Reverse the process and go the opposite direction crossing the left foot over the right.

To assess coordination, the simple act of catching a ball with a friend will help determine coordination level, not to mention the additional benefit of helping to prevent Alzheimer's through social activity. Alone, one can throw the ball against a wall and catch it on the bounce back. Play a game of jacks. Try ping-pong. All these are hand-eye coordination exercises.

Balance and coordination exercises will keep one young and alert for a longer period.

BLOOD CLOTTING

Blood clotting is an important physiological mechanism. If a blood vessel is injured, blood cells and fibrin strands form a clump at the site of injury to stop bleeding. Without this mechanism, we could bleed to death from a simple cut.

Clots can form in the veins of the legs when blood flow slows from inactivity induced by sitting for long periods and failing to exercise. If these clots break off and travel to the heart or lung, it may be fatal if the clot is large enough. That is why long air travel can be dangerous. This danger increases in the obese as the excess fat can squeeze the arteries and veins slowing blood flow even further.

Those at highest risk for blood clots are:
- Smokers
- Those who are bedridden
- The elderly
- Women on birth control pills
- Cancer patients, because they produce chemicals that promote greater platelet production. Platelets are blood cells that play a principle and early role in causing blood to clot

Those patients who fall into any of the categories above should exercise if possible.

A recent study presented at an American Heart Association meeting found that a blood clot dissolver produced by the body, known as tissue type plasminogen activator (t-PA) is thirty percent lower in obese than lean men. However, once the men started an exercise program, the obese men had their levels increased to match the lean men. The conclusion was that regular aerobic exercise would reduce the tendency to clot.

Another study done in the Netherlands on 7,860 people confirmed the above. Understand that the exercise should not be strenuous, because strenuous exercise—with its tendency for injury—may increase the risk for blood clots.

BLOOD PRESSURE

Exercise and one's blood pressure are inversely proportional. In other words the more one exercises the better (lower) one's resting blood pressure may be. One hundred and twenty over eighty (120/80) is a normal reading. The top number is systolic blood pressure, (the pressure in arteries as the ventricles of the heart pumps), and the bottom number is diastolic blood pressure, (the pressure in arteries as the ventricles of the heart are in their resting and filling stage).

Blood pressure has a tendency to increase as one ages. Exercise can prevent that increase. One does not have to run a marathon; walking for one-half hour at least three times per week may be enough. Of course, the more one exercises the better. Any aerobic exercise will do. Get in the habit of walking rather than riding. Take the stairs instead of the elevator. Mow the lawn. A physician should advise you.

If already diagnosed with high blood pressure (hypertension), physician directed exercise would lower it on the average of five to ten points. If that is not enough, blood pressure medication will be necessary.

Why does exercise keep blood pressure in the healthy range and how does it reduce blood pressure that is above the normal range? Regular physical exercise strengthens the heart. Just as a stronger biceps muscle can lift a heavy weight with less effort, so too does a stronger heart muscle pump blood with less effort. This decreases the force within arteries, lowering the blood pressure. It will take at least one month for this benefit to become apparent. The benefits will persist as long as the exercise continues. An additional benefit is that regular exercise (with proper eating, of course) will keep weight down and this will also help to keep blood pressure normal.

A physician must approve an exercise program if one falls into one or more of the following categories:

Someone with a family history of heart problems

If older than forty years of age for a man and fifty years of age for a woman

If the individual is overweight

If the individual is a smoker

If the patient is diagnosed as having hypertension or an elevated cholesterol

When the individual experiences any chest or arm pain or dizziness with exertion

Note that in this section the book has been speaking of aerobic or cardiovascular exercise. Physician approval is also necessary for strength exercises because strength exercises, or heavy lifting when holding one's breath, can raise blood pressure and may not be appropriate for everyone.

Always start an exercise program in a gradual manner and build it up gradually as well. Make enough time for a warm up and cool down before and after exercising.

While exercising, if any one of the following symptoms is experienced, seek immediate medical care:

- Chest, arm, jaw, neck, or upper abdominal pain
- Dizziness
- Irregular heartbeat
- Severe shortness of breath
- Excessive fatigue

BONES

Just as its steel framework holds up a building, bones hold our body up. The steel framework is static—bones are not. The bones of birth are not the bones possessed today.

Osteoblasts are cells that bring calcium into bones to strengthen them. Osteoclasts are cells that take calcium from bones. There is a constant turnover. Lack of exercise slows osteoblastic activity, which results in less calcium delivery and weaker bones. Failure to ingest foods with calcium will have a similar effect.

An exercise must be weight bearing or strength training in order to promote bone strength by stimulating bone formation. Swimming is a great cardiovascular fitness exercise, but is not a weight bearing exercise. Walking, running, tennis, basketball and weight lifting are weight bearing. These exercises, if done with a doctor's approval, will promote bone growth and strength.

Keep in mind that the bone strengthened by exercise is site-specific. If one runs, the leg bones will become stronger. If one lifts weights while standing, the arm and leg bones will both increase in strength. If one does arm curls while sitting down the arm bones will benefit.

The benefits will last only as long as the exercise continues on a regular basis. Age is no barrier. Even at age ninety, bone strength increases with exercise.

Why is this important? Weight bearing exercises prevent osteoporosis, which means porous bone. Bone thins over time, becoming more brittle. The entire process is asymptomatic and fracture may be the first manifestation of the disease.

Bones can become so brittle that even a sneeze, a cough,

bending over, or the simple act of lifting something may cause it to break. The hip, spine and wrist are the most common fractures, but every bone has the potential for injury.

Osteoporosis affects 28,000,000 Americans and is responsible for 1,500,000 fractures per year.

Osteoporosis affects women much more than men.

The reason for the brittleness is the gradual loss of calcium from bone.

Exercise and calcium ingestion are the main preventive measures.

Too much exercise can decrease certain hormones that are necessary for good bone health. Some very well trained women athletes stop menstruating and this may increase the risk of osteoporosis.

With increasing age, keep in mind that regular exercise and calcium rich foods are the key to preventing osteoporosis.

CANCER

Research shows that certain risk factors can increase the chance of getting cancer. The good news is that most people who have the risk factors do not develop cancer, but it can not be known who will be lucky enough to avoid cancer, so learn about the risk factors and avoid those that you can.

The most common risk factors for cancer are:
- Positive family history
- Chemicals
- Viruses and bacteria
- Ionizing radiation
- Hormones
- Obesity
- Poor diet
- Lack of exercise
- Sunlight
- Alcohol
- Tobacco

Poor diet, obesity and tobacco are responsible for the greatest majority of all cancers. Thousands of studies over the years have allowed researchers to publish firm data on cancer risk. Let us take them one at a time.

DIET:
Red meat is incriminated in the cause of colorectal cancer, and demonstrates a probable correlation with endometrial, pancreatic, lung and esophageal cancer.

Why is a natural food cancer producing? At first it was thought that the culprit was herbicides used in cattle feed, but it has since been learned that when the meat is cooked beyond 350 degrees, the amino acids—building blocks of protein—combine with creatine or creatinine (used for energy in muscle) to form substances known as heterocyclic amines (HCA). The higher the temperature, the drier the meat gets, and it is this dry meat that has eight to twelve times as many HCAs as medium cooked meat. Scientists have identified about twenty HCAs in cooked meat. Since HCAs cause colon, breast and prostate cancer in laboratory animals, the International Agency for Research on Cancer has stated that there is a reasonable certainty that it will affect humans the same way. The only way to prove this would be to do research by giving people a heavy diet of very dry very well done meat and see how many get cancer. Of course that is not possible, so scientists do research based upon what people say they eat and then determine whether they get cancer.

Processed meat includes hot dogs, bacon, sausage, beef jerky, sandwich meat, and frozen products with red meat, pastrami and pepperoni. The word processed means that their preparation includes the use of sodium nitrate to keep the meat red and fresh appearing. Sodium nitrate becomes nitrosamines in the body, and this substance promotes cancer. Processed meats are incriminated in colorectal cancer and demonstrate a probable correlation to prostate, stomach, lung and esophageal cancer.

Excessive Calcium rich diets demonstrate a probable correlation with prostate cancer.

Salt heavy diet correlates with a probable increased risk for stomach cancer.

Alcohol, even as little as a drink or two a day, correlates with pre and postmenopausal breast cancer, colorectal cancer, esophageal and lung cancer, and has demonstrated a probable correlation with liver cancer.

Obesity correlates with esophageal, kidney, endometrial, postmenopausal breast cancer, colorectal cancer, and pancreatic cancer, and demonstrates a probable correlation with liver and gallbladder cancer.

It is interesting to note that *increased physical activity* correlates with a decreased risk for colorectal cancer, and a probable decreased risk for breast, endometrial, pancreas and lung cancer.

Also, *breast feeding* correlates with a reduced breast cancer risk and a probable reduction in ovarian cancer risk.

Tobacco causes many cancers, including lung, throat, larynx, mouth, esophagus, colon, bladder, cervix, kidney and pancreas. Prior to 1900, there were no cigarette smokers in the United States. Lung cancer was such a rare disease that when physicians discovered a case, they would report it in medical journals as a rare curiosity. Twenty years later, by 1920, lung cancer began appearing in surprising numbers in men. What once was a rare disease suddenly became common and rose to be the number one cancer in men.

Women did not get lung cancer at this point, but by 1920, they started the smoking habit. Sure enough, by 1940, they too joined the ranks of lung cancer victims.

Wouldn't it be wonderful if everyone practiced preventive medicine by taking all the above statistics to heart and following them to the letter? Ultimately, one's health is in their hands and is dependant on life style changes. Always consult a physician before making any drastic changes.

Now, what is cancer?

A human body has billions of cells. Some say trillions of cells. Billions means a number greater than one followed by nine zeros. Trillions means a number greater than one followed by twelve zeros. Whatever the truth, that is a lot of cells.

Even though our growth stops, many body cells continue to grow and multiply by dividing into two daughter cells known as mitosis. This provides new cells that replace the worn-out cells allowing cellular equilibrium and the ability to enjoy good health.

These billions or trillions of cells all enter what is known as a cell cycle, and in this cell cycle there are built-in controls that determine how fast and when a cell will divide. As soon as there are enough daughter cells made to replace the worn out cells, the cell leaves the cell cycle. Each of our cells has, within its nucleus a pair of signals telling the cells to continue to divide; or stop dividing and exit the cycle. In this way, the body maintains the correct balance of healthy cells.

The nucleus or instruction manual in each cell consists of a DNA molecule, and the information in the manual is in separate "chapters." Each of the chapters contains small paragraphs called GENES, and there are about 24,000 genes in each human cell. The genes work their magic by making proteins—each with a unique function—and it is these proteins that carry out the work of the genes. Genes are the basic units of heredity. Some protect us from cancer and others contribute to cancer development.

A mutation is a change in a gene, and when a gene changes it makes a protein that does not function as it should, so, in many instances, it may lead to a specific disease passed on from parents to offspring. These are hereditary diseases, and are the cause of five to ten percent of cancers.

There is also an acquired mutation caused by environmental factors. They are not hereditary and can not be passed on to children because they are not part of the reproductive cells, but rather are changes in a specific cell and only found in the daughter cells of that cell line.

There are two main genes that play a role in cancer development: oncogenes and tumor suppressor genes:

Oncogenes are a mutation of a normal gene called a proto-oncogene. They control how often a cell divides, but when this normal gene mutates and becomes an oncogene, it operates non-stop. The cell divides too fast and that could lead to cancer. It is as if the gas pedal on an automobile was stuck in the down position and the car cannot stop. Geneticists have discovered one-hundred oncogenes.

Tumor suppressor genes are genes that keep cell division running at the appropriate slow pace. They also repair DNA mistakes made when cells divide, and if the mistake is too great, order the cell to commit suicide by a process known as apoptosis or programmed cell death. When the tumor suppressor gene is defective, cells grow at an uncontrolled rate, which leads to cancer. A tumor suppressor gene that keeps the cell from dividing too fast is like the brake pedal of a car, which slows the car down. Geneticists have discovered thirty tumor suppressor genes.

Note that there is a difference between these two types of genes. The oncogene is an activated proto-oncogene, and the tumor suppressor gene is an inactivated, or turned off gene. The majority of oncogenes are acquired mutations, and tumor suppressor genes can be hereditary or acquired. The good news is that research has led to some cancer cures and there are hopes for many more. Based upon current research advances, there is an ever-increasing optimism about cancer cure. Time will tell if the optimistic forecasts are accurate.

CARDIAC DISEASE

The cardiac disease referred to is coronary artery disease (coronary atherosclerosis). Coronary refers to arteries of the heart, and the word atherosclerosis is of Greek origin: *athero* meaning pasty gruel, and *sclerosis* meaning hardness. So atherosclerosis is a process where fatty material, cholesterol, calcium, various cellular waste materials and other products build up in the heart arteries' inner lining forming a substance called plaque. A sudden rupture of this plaque can cause the artery to obstruct resulting in the disruption of blood flow to a portion of the heart muscle. If the artery is small enough, the block can cause a heart attack—the death of a portion of the heart muscle, and if large enough will cause the death of the patient.

What this means is that the first symptom of coronary atherosclerosis may be quick death, so paying attention to the risk factors that can lead to this sudden, unexpected end is prudent.

The risk factors for coronary artery disease are obesity, elevated blood pressure, elevated cholesterol, smoking, diabetes and lack of exercise. Inactive people have double the risk of heart disease. How does exercise help?

- Burning calories by exercise causes weight reduction and the less one weighs the less the chance of heart disease
- Exercise will lower LDL cholesterol ("bad" cholesterol), and elevate HDL cholesterol ("good" cholesterol)
- Exercise will lower both systolic and diastolic blood pressure

CARDIAC OUTPUT, STROKE VOLUME AND HEART RATE

The heart muscle (cardiac muscle) is a different muscle than the muscles that cover and attach to our skeletons (skeletal muscle). Cardiac muscle's purpose is endurance. After all, what other muscle can perform on a continuous basis for 80 plus years? Each cubic millimeter of heart muscle has 2000 capillaries (tiny blood vessels between the arteries and veins) designed to deliver blood (with its oxygen) to itself without letup. With exercise, the heart muscle gets a bit bigger. It acquires a bigger **stroke volume**. Stroke volume is the volume of blood that the left ventricle ejects to the entire body with each beat.

At rest, our heart is beating at an average of seventy beats per minute. With each beat, the heart pumps out about seventy milliliters of blood. This amounts to roughly five liters of blood per minute for a healthy resting **cardiac output.**

With exercise, the resting **heart rate** may decrease, but at the same time, its efficiency increases to the extent that it will now deliver about 90 ml per minute, as opposed to the average 70 ml per beat.

What has happened is that the heart has become more efficient. It now performs the same work with less beats and less cardiac muscle energy demand. This means the heart is stronger, a benefit which affects the entire body.

CARTILAGE

Cartilage is a protein that acts as a cushion between the bones of a joint. Osteoarthritis, or degenerative arthritis, results from the breakdown of cartilage in our joints. At least twenty million people in the United States suffer from osteoarthritis. It is more common in males under age forty-five and in females after age fifty-five. It affects the spine, hands, feet, and weight bearing joints such as the knee and hip. The prevailing theory was that exercise will aggravate cartilage destruction thus worsening osteoarthritis—but a recent study has changed this perception.

Two researchers in Sweden recruited forty-five people between the age of thirty-five and fifty who had knee meniscus repair and were thus prime candidates for future development of osteoarthritis. They randomized them to an "exercise" or a "no exercise" group. One group did aerobic and weight bearing exercises for one hour three times per week for four months. MRI scans measured a specific chemical in cartilage that determined its strength and elasticity.

In the "exercise" group, many more reported improved symptoms and gains in physical activity than in the "no exercise" group. In addition, the improvements in the MRIs showed a strong correlation with the increased exercise.

The conclusion was that cartilage responds well to exercise, similar to the responses expressed by bone and muscle.

COLLATERAL CIRCULATION

When an artery to any part of the body becomes blocked, how does blood get to the affected part? The answer is via collateral circulation. Imagine what the flow of traffic would be on a busy street if there were no detours available to get around cumbersome construction.

The body, in its wisdom, recognizes the blockage and promotes the development of small blood vessels (angiogenesis) that go past the block to bring blood and oxygen to that portion of the body supplied by the blocked artery.

Aerobic exercises enhance this crucial mechanism. That is a proven fact.

Imagine the importance of this when it comes to coronary artery circulation (blood traffic flow). The exercise-induced formation of new coronary arteries prevent the heart attack from developing.

DEPRESSION

Exercise is as effective in treating depression as antidepressants, individual psychotherapy and group psychotherapy. Numerous studies have proven this.

What kinds of exercise will be effective? The principle one is walking, and the good news is that it brings rapid relief even within ten minutes after one study.

If effective at all, medications will take at least two to three weeks to show improvement. One of the side effects of some anti depressants, however, is suicide. Close monitoring is essential for some patients who choose this route.

The effects of exercise as therapy will be long lasting. In one exercise study, walking every day for seven weeks improved mood for five months. The exercises are aerobic and include walking, swimming and bicycling. Another study demonstrated that exercise results in improvement for as long as the exercising continues. Remember also that exercise has none of the side effects that are so common in antidepressants.

Studies done on children through old age have shown that all age groups benefit. Not only do depressive symptoms improve, but also there is more vigor, less fatigue, less anxiety, less confusion, less stress, better integration with peers and improved mental functioning.

How does exercise account for this improvement? Through endorphins, adrenaline, serotonin and dopamine. These are powerful hormone-like substances produced in the brain that work together and promote a state of well being and a sense of accomplishment, even to the point of euphoria in some instances. Endorphins can even mask pain to the extent that one will exercise through the injury causing further problems.

So listen to what your body tells you and check out any injury.

In general, if depressed seek medical attention, and remember that exercise can be an important component of therapy so long as your physician approves.

DIABETES MELLITUS

The hormone Insulin, a protein secreted by islet cells in the pancreas, controls blood sugar. The pancreas is an organ situated behind the stomach and has many functions including making digestive enzymes and hormones. Carbohydrates (sugars) are absorbed into the blood stream from the small intestine after a meal. As the sugar in the blood rises, the pancreas will secrete more insulin to push the sugars into the cells of the body for energy use. When this system works well the blood sugar balance stays within the normal range.

An elevated blood sugar level indicates Diabetes Mellitus, a malfunction of the above normal mechanism.

Type 1 diabetes affects younger patients and is an autoimmune disease. Viewing the islet cells as foreign, the immune system destroys these insulin-producing cells of the pancreas resulting in the inability to make sufficient insulin. This condition requires daily insulin injections to stay healthy.

Type 2 diabetes is a condition resulting from the decreased ability of the body to process sugar. This condition is increasing because it results from obesity, which is on the rise and causes a condition known as insulin resistance: the body becomes resistant to insulin's effects. In other words, the insulin stops working as well in an effort by the body to deliver less sugar to muscles and fat, an attempt to reduce the obesity trend. As insulin put less sugar into the cells, the sugar becomes elevated in the blood stream causing pre-diabetes or a full-blown diabetic state.

A fasting blood sugar level of 100 to 125mg/dl on two occasions confirms the diagnosis of pre-diabetes. Another test, HemoglobinA1C, or the level of sugar carried in the hemoglobin molecule, measures blood sugar levels over the last three months. This is a form of red blood cell hemoglobin combined with glucose and should not exceed more than about six percent of all hemoglobin. The HemoglobinA1C, originally developed as a means to evaluate diabetic control, is also useful to diagnose diabetes.

Gestational diabetes is the diabetes of pregnancy. It puts a woman at higher risk for pregnancy complications, and it often resolves after birth. Women diagnosed with this condition should keep their weight in check to prevent pre or full-blown diabetes after delivery.

The control of diabetes depends upon a compliant, educated patient working in conjunction with a dedicated healthcare team.

About 30 million people in the United States have type-2 diabetes, which is associated with lack of exercise, obesity and genetics.

The bad news is that the high blood sugar levels associated with diabetes damage blood vessels leading to diffuse vascular disease including heart disease, stroke, kidney disease and blindness.

In a study done by Canadian researchers, two hundred and fifty sedentary Canadian diabetics made up four different groups:

1. No exercise
2. Forty-five minutes of aerobic exercise three times a week
3. Forty-five minutes of strength exercises three times per week
4. Forty-five minutes of both aerobic and strength exercises three times per week

The conclusion the Canadian researchers came to is that exercising can lower A1C. Aerobic activity burns calories and strengthens the vascular system, including the heart. Strength training improves muscle strength and makes the muscles more sensitive to the effects of insulin. Physician approval for any type of exercise in a diabetic is mandatory.

Exercise can lower A1C as well as any medication used today for diabetes, although medication works best when supplemented with exercise.

DIGESTION

The digestive system organs (stomach, small intestine, large intestine, pancreas, liver and gall bladder) function as a team to help the body break down food into small nutrient molecules that can be absorbed into the blood stream for delivery to all the cells of the body. If the system malfunctions, digestive problems occur.

One digestive problem is constipation defined as infrequent or difficult passage of stools, hard stools and a feeling of incomplete evacuation. A common cause is the lack of fiber in the diet and an absence of physical activity. The solution, therefore, is high fiber foods such as whole grain breads, high fiber cereals, beans, fresh fruits and vegetables, and light, low impact exercise done on a regular basis. A result of exercise, as far as the digestive tract is concerned, is a stronger and more regular contraction of the intestinal muscles. In addition, the combination of the dietary modification and the exercises should alleviate constipation unless there are more serious causes (and there often are), so medical consultation is mandatory.

Another problem that can be relieved by exercise is heartburn. However, some heartburn is due to gastro esophageal reflux disease, a condition where acid in the stomach migrates back up the esophagus causing the burning symptom. If left untreated, this condition can result in esophageal inflammation or esophageal cancer. Therefore, once again, medical consultation is necessary.

Remember to wait at least two hours after a meal to exercise.

ENDOMETRIOSIS

The endometrium is the name for the cells that line the uterus. These cells belong nowhere else. Endometriosis is a medical condition where the uterine lining cells also grow outside of the uterus, on fallopian tubes, ovaries or tissue lining the pelvis. Even though the endometrial cells are outside of the body of the uterus, they still react as if they were in the uterus and they bleed each month, irritating the surrounding tissue.

Researchers have determined that aerobic exercises such as jogging, bicycling or skating at least three times a week for one-half hour can reduce the risk of endometriosis by two-thirds.

In addition, exercise raises endorphin levels that promote endometriosis pain relief and reduce estrogen levels that have the effect of reducing pain as well. Therefore, exercise has a dual effect: it not only helps prevents endometriosis, but relieves symptoms as well.

Alcohol and caffeine raise estrogen levels. Women with endometriosis should avoid these substances.

HDL

The book has discussed HDL cholesterol in a previous section, but it is so important that it merits further discussion.

HDL cholesterol, also known as good cholesterol, pulls cholesterol off the artery walls. Cholesterol and other substances form plaque that blocks arteries and causes heart attacks, peripheral artery disease or strokes. It takes this excess cholesterol back to the liver for processing, which can then excrete cholesterol from the body.

HDL cholesterol lower than 40 carries with it a greater risk for coronary artery disease. A level of 60 or greater is protective against artery disease. In fact, the higher the better.

Aerobic exercise will raise HDL levels and the longer one exercises the greater the HDL increase. There are also other ways to raise HDL:

- Lose weight
- Remove Trans-fats from the diet
- Stop smoking
- Get recommended amount of fiber (25 g/day according to the FDA).
- Increase monounsaturated fat in the diet (olive oil, canola oil, peanut butter)
- Eat fish with omega 3 fatty acids

IMMUNE SYSTEM

We owe a state of good health to our immune system; it is a collaborative mechanism that protects us from disease by utilizing a sophisticated team of specialized organs and cells that differentiate self from non-self. This ability is important because every body cell carries distinctive molecules on their surfaces that identify it as **self**. Recognizing this self-marker, immune cells (white blood cells) coexist with body cells in a state known as self-tolerance. However, predators that attack our body—bacteria, viruses, fungi, parasites, cancer cells and transplanted organs—that do not carry this self-marker will find themselves subjected to a vigorous assault by the immune system.

There you have it—a one-paragraph summary of a subject that could take ten volumes to describe. Needless to say, a healthy immune system is vital for good health.

Moderate, consistent exercise boosts immunity over the long-term. It boosts the production of immune system cells. Exercise protects us from acquiring upper respiratory infections. During exercise, immune cells circulate through the body faster and are better able to kill bacteria and viruses. After exercise, the immune system returns to normal, but consistent exercise improves functioning for a longer period. The key is moderation and consistency.

Intense exercise will cause a reduction in immunity for up to three days after the intense physical exertion. This is because the body produces certain hormones that lower immunity for a short period. Therefore, if you are a tri-athlete or a marathon runner it is important to rest for a few days after competition.

Physical stress—and psychological stress—promote the release of the stress hormones cortisol and adrenaline. These hormones raise blood pressure and suppress the immune system. University researchers evaluated the caretakers of Alzheimer's patients and found that they had twice the occurrence of upper respiratory infections as non-caregivers.

Regular, moderate exercise will keep the immune system healthy.

LONGEVITY

There have been enough studies done to make a definite assertion about exercise: It increases longevity. Records of more than 5,000 older and middle-aged individuals showed that those with moderate levels of exercise (defined as walking for thirty minutes a day five days per week), lived 1.3 to 1.5 years longer. In addition, those who engaged in vigorous exercise defined as running for half an hour per day five days per week, lived 3.5 to 3.7 years longer.

There is no doubt that exercise adds years and enhances quality of life. It is never too late to start. Check with a physician and with approval—get moving.

LYMPHEDEMA

Let us start with an anatomical review:

Within our arteries is blood. Plasma is the fluid part of the blood.

Capillaries are tiny microscopic arteries. When the fluid plasma leaves the capillaries to enter the tissue spaces, the fluid's name changes to interstitial fluid.

When the interstitial fluid enters the lymph channels, the fluid's name changes to lymph.

These lymph channels enlarge further and become lymph ducts that deposit the lymph back to the blood vessel circulation (veins) near the heart. Once back into the blood circulation the name of he fluid reverts to plasma.

There are lymph glands along the course of the lymph channels. The purpose of these lymph glands is to act as a filter of foreign substances (bacteria, viruses) from the lymph as it makes its way back to the blood vessel circulation.

If there is disruption of lymph circulation, it can cause arm swelling known as lymphedema. If a woman has a mastectomy with removal of the lymph nodes under the arm, or has had surgery or radiation therapy or both, these therapies can also disrupt the lymph circulation and swelling of the arm may result.

For many years, physicians have instructed their mastectomy patients to avoid any lifting with the affected arm, fearing that the swelling will increase. This has changed.

A new study, randomized to include half of the women doing weight training with the affected arm and half the women doing no exercise, demonstrated that the women who exercised had a significant decrease in the amount of swelling in the affected arm as well as greater strength in that arm.

METABOLISM

We all need energy (calories) to live. We use these calories when exercising, sleeping, and eating. Metabolism is the number of calories used to maintain body functions.

Muscle needs more calories to function than fat does. Therefore, the more muscle in relation to fat, the higher the metabolism.

Symptoms of a slow metabolism include a feeling of coldness, fatigue, dry skin, constipation, slow pulse and low blood pressure. However, there are medical conditions such as an under active thyroid that can cause a slow metabolism. Therefore, check with a physician in order to be sure to rule out a medical problem.

Here are some metabolism facts:
- The greater the muscle mass the faster the metabolism
- When metabolism slows, the body will convert calories to fat
- Women have slower metabolism than men—due to estrogen
- Men have faster metabolism than women—due to testosterone
- Metabolism slows down as we age
- Antidepressant medication can slow down metabolism
- Regular moderate exercise will speed up metabolism
- Any illness can slow metabolism

Muscle mass can be increased by weight and strength exercises. Aerobic exercise reduces fat. The net result will be to increase metabolism and body function will improve.

MUSCLE TONE, STRENGTH AND ENDURANCE

Muscle tone equals firmness. Muscle strength refers to the greatest amount of force a muscle can exert. Muscle endurance refers to how long a muscle can stay in a state of contraction.

Before embarking on a program to build up muscles, one needs medical clearance. These exercises are for motivated and healthy individuals. They include calisthenics (push-ups, abdominal crunches, etc), stretch bands, weight machines and hand weights.

An individual's fitness level is first determined to know where to start. As always, get medical clearance from a physician.

Besides the good effect on muscles, exercise will also:
- Sculpt the body
- Strengthen bones
- Improve posture
- Increase metabolism
- Elevate mood and your sense of self-worth
- Improve appearance

SKIN

By increasing circulation, exercise delivers vital nutrients to skin cells and removes toxins from skin cells. This provides optimal conditions for the skin to make vital collagen—the building block support for wrinkle-free skin.

For those with an acne problem, exercise reduces stress, and with stress reduction there is less adrenal gland production of testosterone-like hormones, which can aggravate acne. In addition, reduction of these hormones may reduce or slow hair loss.

Exercise also increases sweating, which has the benefit of unplugging pores, thereby helping to improve acne and reduce flare-ups.

Overall, an optimal complexion results when skin health improves.

SLEEP

The National Sleep Foundation states that a regular aerobic exercise regimen will result in better sleep. Sleep deprivation is a major cause of accidents and poor work performance.

A team from Northwestern University in Evanston, Illinois funded by the National Institute on Aging, studied twenty-three sedentary adults aged fifty-five and older who had trouble either falling or staying asleep. One group exercised on a treadmill or stationary bicycle. Another group did not exercise, but participated in cooking classes or trips to museums.

The conclusion was that those that exercised had a significant improvement in the quality of their sleep, fewer symptoms of depression, a better mood and enhanced alertness and vitality

STRESS

The World Book Encyclopedia defines stress as pressure, force, strain. In 1936, Hans Selye, a pioneer researcher, defined stress as "the non-specific response of the body to any demand for change." He experimented with animals, subjecting them to unpleasant physical and emotional stimuli and noted the consequences including adrenal gland enlargement, stomach ulcers and shrunken lymphoid tissue. In addition, he found that these animals developed similar diseases to that seen in human beings including heart attack and stroke. Also seen in humans are depression, sleep problems, memory deficits, digestive problems and eczema.

A simple definition of stress is difficult because what is stress for one individual is not for the next. It is a variable phenomenon and affects each of us differently, but if stress is a constant companion, serious health consequences can result.

Physiologically, stress induces the hypothalamus of the brain located at the base of the brain to set off an alarm in the form of nerve and hormonal signals that result in the adrenal gland liberating both cortisone and adrenaline. The net affect is to elevate blood pressure, increase heart rate, increase blood sugar and increase body repair—all preparing the body for a flight or fight response while at the same time suppressing other functions unnecessary during stressful times such as digestion, reproduction and growth.

If a person is under continuous stress and knows it, there is nothing better than exercise to relieve stress and reset the body's physiological response to normal. Any exercise preferred and approved by a physician can relieve stress. It works by increasing endorphin production from the brain, it improves mood, depression and anxiety, steers mental focus inward, promotes better sleep and can help to promote a sense of calmness.

Physical activity is one of the best methods to combat stress.

TRIGLYCERIDES

There are two sources of triglyceride (blood fats): eating fatty foods and converting carbohydrate to fat in the liver.

Too much triglyceride in the blood can cause atherosclerosis, promote blood clotting, and can cause pancreatitis, a serious inflammation of the pancreas.

One critical aspect of an elevated triglyceride is that it is often associated with other abnormalities including low HDL, high LDL, abdominal obesity (potbelly) elevated blood pressure, insulin resistance and type 2 diabetes mellitus. Metabolic syndrome is the name for this collection of findings. Those who develop this syndrome are prone to coronary artery disease and diabetes.

Insulin resistance is critical for the development of this syndrome. One of the main functions of insulin is to store fat in body fat cells and muscle cells and allow entry of sugar into cells. The American diet on top of a lack of exercise promotes this fattening effect and, as mentioned before, gaining weight reduces the efficiency of insulin. As the efficiency of insulin decreases, less glucose can get in to body cells for energy and therefore glucose levels elevate in the blood stream resulting in a pre-diabetic or diabetic state.

Those who have this syndrome (about 30 percent of the American population) have double the risk of heart disease and four times the risk of diabetes mellitus.

Exercise and weight loss will reverse the metabolic syndrome thus lowering cardiac risk. In more severe cases, medication may also be necessary.

UPPER RESPIRATORY INFECTIONS

In the fall of 2008, 1002 men and women, aged eighteen to eighty-five, were involved in an experiment correlating upper respiratory infection rates with level of exercise performed every week.

The conclusion: The participants in the study who were physically fit and who exercised more than five times per week had about half as many upper respiratory infections as those who reported less physical activity. In addition, those who exercised also experienced less upper respiratory symptoms.

The British journal of sports medicine concluded, "Working out on a regular schedule will help ward off colds and flu." This is because exercise strengthens the immune system and also improves lung function.

VARICOSE VEINS

Veins carry deoxygenated blood to the right side of the heart for delivery to the lungs where the blood picks up oxygen (the one exception to this is oxygenated blood carried by pulmonary veins from the lung to the left side of the heart for deliver to the body.

Veins have valves within them that prevent blood from backing up. When the valves become defective, they do not close well and blood backs up widening and accentuating the veins. The name for this anatomical defect is varicose veins (widened, blood-filled veins).

Varicose veins may be due to a genetic problem, obesity, pregnancy, heart disease, or abdominal tumors.

Exercise is effective in causing leg muscles to contract (running, walking, bicycling) thus squeezing the blood on to the heart and helping to prevent the blood backup that can aggravate the varicose veins. It is not necessary to treat most varicose veins. Check with a physician if severe pain develops in varicose veins as it could mean a clot has developed.

WEIGHT CONTROL

Weight depends upon the amount of calories ingested minus the amount burned. Burning less than ingested will result in the excess calories deposited as fat, adding weight to the body. If one burns more than ingested, weight will decrease.

Since regular exercise burns calories, it is an effective way to reduce fat stores (accompanied by a sensible diet, of course.). So, exercise and sensible calorie reduction is more effective than just dieting.

There it is; the world's number one prescription—The Perfect Prescription—Exercise. If taken with medical supervision it is safe and free of the specific side effects that come with every prescription drug. It does not treat only one problem, it treats almost all organ systems and results in good health, better mood, increased longevity plus all the other pearls you just learned. No prescription medicine can equal the versatility, the depth, the power of exercise. Where will you ever get a prescription to equal it? You cannot. So see a physician, get a complete history and physical examination and risk factor analysis. Practice early detection and prevention, and, once granted permission, do some regular exercises—for the rest of your life.

We cannot help but be impressed by the clinical acumen and the genius of the ancients who, in the days before research and clinical trials and based upon their own observations, could come up with the wisdom as exemplified below.

"As long as a person exercises and exerts himself...sickness does not befall him and his strength increases... But one who is idle and does not exercise...even if he eats healthy foods and maintains healthy habits, all his days will be of ailment and his strength will diminish."

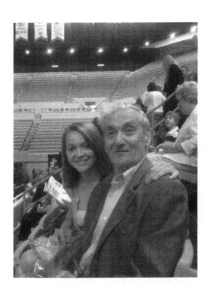

A graduate of the University of Illinois College of Medicine, Sheldon Cohen has practiced Internal Medicine, served as a medical director of a Chicago area Catholic Hospital and two Health Maintenance Organizations, taught physical diagnosis and internal medicine at two Chicago area medical schools, served as a quality consultant for hospitals in the United States, Europe and South America, served as a consultant to the Ministry of Health in Ukraine, lectures to lay audiences on medical topics and is the author of twelve books.

Megan Godwin was born on June 12, 1990 in Frankfort, Germany. Raised in Tulsa, Oklahoma, she graduated from Jenks high school in 2008 and currently attends the University of Oklahoma where she majors in health and exercise science and minors in zoology and chemistry. She is eternally grateful for the love and support that she receives from her grandparents, her mother, Gail Cohen, and her father, Gary Godwin. After graduation, she would like to attend medical school and is currently undecided on her focus.